Arresting Cancer Organically

This worked for my mum it may work for you.
Relief For Cancer Victims.

By Robyn Ji Smith

Edition 3a

ISBN:9798387058288 *For Paper Back Copy*

Independent Publisher Beauty Pathways Academy at

Beauty School Books

Copyright 2009

Copyright

Watch Movies That Make You Laugh.

Index

It is my hope that this brief story will give Cancer suffers extra energetic years. When they have been told their Cancer is progressing rapidly and nothing can be done - try this. My mother was given a few weeks to live and I was not ready to lose my mother. This white witch craft cure, gave my mother and I the time we needed and definitely amazingly returned her quality of life. However now days my family and I, no longer are called witches as we have certificates in Clinical Aromatherapy and Reiki.

Will this organic recipe help everyone? I do not know. Does it cure cancer , on a cellular level I do not know that either . But -what I do know you are about to find out. This cure helped my mum regain her quality of life and it may help you or someone you love. When mum was given three weeks or less to live, she looked like a dead man walking. Her skin tone was a dirty grey tone., She was passing out, having trouble eating, in a lot of pain and sleeping more than normal. She had not been offered a nurse, nor pain relief.

Before The Cancer Notification

This is a little about us and the neglect or lack of medical knowledge of general practitioners.

My life was about to bloom, so I thought. I was preparing to retire I bought a caravan, a four wheel drive, solar panels, a free campsite directory and mum and I were going to do some more travelling. In June 2006 mum and I left for Queensland I was going to spend six months with my son and four grandchildren. Mum was going to stay for a month, then return home. At the end of my stay, mum was to return to the Gold Coast in Queensland and we were to continue our adventure.

During the time mum and I were at my sons, I noticed my mother was having trouble eating and keeping her food down. Thinking it may be an allergic reaction to dairy, I tried to encourage her to use either rice or soy milk in her coffee. No way was she going to change; mum loved her full cream milk coffee and was not even going to dilute the milk with some water. She would not come to the doctors with me and kept insisting she would see her doctor when she returned home. Our trip to Queensland we toured the outback and as I owned land in Burren Junction we spent a week at the Artesian Bore. The water there is definitely - magical. Mum had been floating for about 30 minutes.

My mother lived in Woy Woy New South Wales. My Daughter has a home about 3 kilometers away from my mum in Umina Beach. My brother and his family also live in Woy Woy about a kilometer from our mum's home.

Watch Movies That Make You Laugh.

The thing that mum has always had that most folk don't seem to understand is :- The importance of is gratitude, the power in words we speak, mindfulness, trust in our higher powers and knowing the difference of good and evil forces here on earth and power foods. Power food cannot be packaged. Power foods walk or grown.

 Mum also ran a positive thinking group at Woy Woy Hospital on Sundays and on Tuesdays in a hall in East Gosford. She had been running these free meetings for over 30 years. Mum decided not to drive anymore. Mum told us the car was getting old and costly to keep on the road. There was no bus to get her to the Sunday meeting and she would need to rely on other people. My good-hearted brother bought her a new bike. He would go to her place and check the tyre pressures for her each week.

Before we went to Queensland mum in her eighties, decided she wanted to ride her push bike to the shops.

Mum fell off her pushbike while peddling home from the shops. Her face was very badly bruised but she said she felt fine. Her Doctor assured us she was fine. But she was not fine she had actually passed out. That was the beginning of mum passing out quite often. Her face healed then one morning we arrived to see her and her face was badly bruised again. Mum had fallen during the night and hit her face on the washing machine. Then the storey unfolded we found out from her meeting friends that they had found her out cold on several occasions over the past five years. Her doctors sent her for tests but found nothing wrong. During one test they forgot to strap her in and she fell as they rotated the bed. Mum laughed and said,

"Well, I must have strong bones I haven't broken any".

A few months after mum return from my sons' home, my daughter rang and said,

"Mum I have to call into check on Nan every morning before work and every night because she is sleeping a lot and forgetting to eat. She is not interested in the garden nor is she keeping the house as clean as she usually does. Nan is always in her nighty and she is wearing the same nighty for days".

 This was so unlike my mother, even as children our mother kept her home spotlessly clean you could eat off her floors any time of the day or night. At that point my daughter changed her job to part time to keep a better eye on her Nan.

In the mean time my son gained week on week off, access to his four children. He was over the moon. However, the private catholic school they were attending was 17 kilometers from his home. Therefore, I needed to stay and help. His ten year old son refused to go back and live with his mum. We leveled the ground on the other side of the creek and set up my caravan, I drove the children to and from school.

A few months later we found mum had gone blind in one eye and she was becoming deaf. After lots of appointments with specialists and many treatments they never found her Cancer.

They did insert a bionic hearing aid (called a cochlear implant) but could do nothing about the loss of sight in her right eye. They also could not work out what to do with her inability to swallow. Mum waited many weeks sometimes months each time her Doctor organized yet another appointment with another Specialist.

 My mother was scheduled for a series of tests. During the next few weeks mum did not comprehend what she was being told nor understood the sea of information she was being given. Mum said, felt fine and was not in any pain. So, she told us all! But we all noticed she had constant head pain.

They do say that Cancer is a silent killer and I now understand that saying. My mother is a gentle natured woman that everyone loves. She never complains but remember the squeaky door does get the most attention. Listen to your higher power. If you have a reoccurring pain have it investigated.

My Mother was told in September 2007 that she had terminal Cancer and that it was very aggressive. The specialist said, she would not see Christmas so to start saying her good byes and to get ready. My mother 82 years of age was at a specialist in North Gosford at the time when she was given this news. That is only a distance of about 16 kilometers from her home. However, to get home she needed to change buses twice and walk two kilometers or catch a taxi or wait an hour for the third bus. Mum had not told any of the family she was going to the specialist that day, she was completely alone when she was told her life was to end within a few weeks and there was nothing that could be done.

Specialist are expensive. Surely, they are making enough money that they could do either a home visit when the Cancer person has family around them or insist she/he come back that day with a family member. But you know, they train for many years so they can earn big bucks and have developed a grand life style. It costs time to be considerate and time is money. A home visit would be a big financial loss for that day. Heaven forbid the Specialist would not be able to buy that $300 bottle of champagne for dinner. Yes, you guessed it we were upset that they told mum in an office far from her home, and when she was alone.

Watch Movies That Make You Laugh.

Later we found out mum had head and stomach pains for over eight years. I have since heard that Cancer actually can take up to 10 years to kill you. It is that most of us do not squeak that door enough. We go on thinking it will pass or it is normal to have things go wrong as we are ageing. They cannot see Cancer in our body with a CT scan they can just see hot pockets. Yet CT scans can detect most forms of cancer and no one had offered my mother a CT scan.

A WARNING ABOUT CT SCANS:

Although they show hot spots that are probably cancer cells, a CT scan gives you unhealthy and dangerous amounts of Radiation. I am guessing that is why they did not give my elderly mother a CT scan.

My daughter (Alisha) immediately gave up her job, Alisha drove mum up to see me. They did not want to give me this devastating news over the telephone. When I looked at mum, I could see she was very ill. How did this happen so quickly? In June she looked fine and now in September she looked like a dead person walking. After talking through her situation with mum I said,

" Mum would you like to live? I know you are saying to us all, that it is your time to go and you are happy to go but I am not ready to lose you".

"Well " mum said, "I would like to live to see Christmas but I am ready to go and I feel like it is my time and I do not have the energy to keep going until Christmas. The Doctors have said, I only have a few weeks".

"Mum will you let me try to help you"?

Watch Movies That Make You Laugh.

"Yes love, if I can see Christmas I will be very happy".

The very next day I went shopping for the essential oil of Lavender distilled in Tasmania. I rang my friend who was a Beauty Therapist but, in her country, she had trained as a herbalist. She told me to research beetroot juice and Turmeric so I did.

I could not bear to lose her so quickly. My mum did not want to have chemotherapy and the doctors said it would not help her due to her age and her cancer was spreading too fast. The main areas of cancer were in her throat and stomach.

. They also explained that Chemo and radiation therapy is sometimes given to reduce the pain but does not always cure Cancer.

I purchased some Turmeric and empty gelatin capsules and made tablets I gave her eight a day for the 1st week then reduced it to four a day. I made her beetroot juice and added other things like apples and oranges, parsley, spinach, ginger, and celery to it.

You can also buy empty plant cellulose capsules. The beetroot and turmeric are the two main healers but turmeric is activated by black pepper so I added pepper to her tablets and encouraged her to have pepper in her coffee.

At the time she had not been able to eat solid food for several months and had been living on milk, custard and smoked Salmon. After several days on the beetroot juice, black pepper and turmeric routine, we could see a big difference in her. She did not gain any weight but she did get colour back in her skin. The deathly grey colour of her skin changed to a beautiful alive looking peaches and cream colour. So, it was wonderful to see her normal colour return. Her headaches persisted but she had energy. She was no longer vomiting every time she something to drink or eat.

Watch Movies That Make You Laugh.

Note in 1994 they discovered that Lavender grown in Tasmania had Cancer healing properties in their essential oil. Then it was all hushed up. I think soon after a chemical company bought out the Lavender farm. I was no longer able to buy oil straight from the farm.

Bath Oil For Cancer Cure

I would encourage mum to put this mix in her bath each day or to rub it onto her body. I made a large bottle of this mix but here is the recipe:-

In 100ml of Olive oil add

30 drops of Lavender oil from Tasmania.

Add 3 drops of pepper essential oil

10 drops of rose geranium essential oil.

5 drops clove oil.

Don't add more drops because you are fearful of losing the one you love. Less is most often best. They must not put this oil directly on their face. Keep this mixture in a glass narrow neck dark bottle, in a dark cool place.

Contra indications to lavender is low blood pressure. If you or your loved one has low blood pressure change lavender oil for Sandalwood, or German chamomile. Or cypress or myrrh. They are also high in sesquiterpenes.

They can massage this oil in every night or put one teaspoon in a foot bath and soak for 25 minutes so the osmosis takes it into the blood.

Watch Movies That Make You Laugh.

Or put 2 tablespoons into a warm bath and soak for 25 minutes.

It is important that they bath or soak by candle light as incandescent lights turn essential oil molecules into toxic vapors. Or they could bath before the sun goes down. But the oils work best of a night. The body pulsates inward after 5pm. During the day the body pulsates outward to rid the body of toxic waste that is why a walk in the sunlight is so important to good health. Geranium is recently been hailed as a cure for cancer that is why it needs to be added to this bath oil mix. Organic germanium is a biological-response modifier. Biological-response modifiers are substances that can enable the body to change its response to tumors. Organic germanium will stimulate the body's immune system, making it potentially effective in the treatment of cancer as well as other degenerative diseases. I have a passion for the use of rose geranium and have seen amazing results in healing sores, wrinkles, boils and many other skin complaints. When you can visually see something working externally you know it is working from the inside out. Essential oils need to be mixed with a carrier oil to penetrate safely into the blood stream.

Essential Oils must never be used neat they are far to strong for our liver to deal with. They must be blended with a base oil. The best essential oils for cancer patients are the oils high in sesquiterpenes.

 My favourite base oil that I mix my essential oils in is Olive oil.

1. Olive Oil Is Rich in Healthy Monounsaturated Fats
2. Olive Oil Has High Antioxidant properties
3. Olive Oil Has Strong Anti-Inflammatory Properties
4. Olive Oil May Help Prevent Strokes
5. Olive Oil Is Protective Against Heart Disease

Watch Movies That Make You Laugh.

6. Olive Oil Is **Not** Associated with Weight Gain and
    Obesity
7. Olive Oil May Fight Alzheimer's Disease

Essential Oil Blending Chart

Blending For Safe Use Of Essential Oils

Carrier Oil For Body	Essential Oil For Body	Carrier Oil For Face	Essential Oil For Face
100 ml	50 drops	100 ml	25 drops
50 ml	25 drops	50 ml	12 to 13 drops
25 ml	12 to 13 drops	25 ml	10 drops
20 ml	10 drops	20 ml	5 drops
10 ml	5 drops	10 ml	2 drops
5 ml	2 drops	5 ml	1 drop

Always Blend in Dark Glass Medicine Bottles
The face and neck skin are thinner and more sensitive than the rest of the body.
Therefore, the mixtures should be at half strength. A general rule blending table.
After choosing the essential oil or a few oils to add to the bend you must follow the contraindication rules for each person.
Body Blending Table.- for the body 2%   Face Blending Table 1%
Aged skin is half the above dose for body use face blending for face blending use half face drop quantity.

Pregnancy Blending Table.

Carrier - Essential Oil for Pregnancy 1/2% (Half a percent).
 after 3rd month
 20 ml Carrier oil/body butter - maximum is 2 drops or less
 30 ml Carrier oil/body butter - maximum is 3 drops or less
 50 ml Carrier oil/body butter - maximum is 5 drops or less
100 ml Carrier oil/body butter - maximum is 10 drops or less

Babies over 6-12 months use half a percent as for pregnancy. We advise not to use essential oils on babies. Use wool fat or bees wax, mixed with olive oil for nappy rash. Warm the wax and blend in the olive oil. Place in a dark glass jar. Place 1 drop only of Lavender EO on their bed under their pillow to calm them.

Post Natal Depression	SNIFF - Rose, Bergamot, Sweet Orange, or Sandalwood And Meditate.
Labour Pains	Clary Sage to start labour Lavender to relax Chamomile to release tension Geranium - to expel afterbirth Sniff Frankincense for fear Sweet Marjoram for spasms
Morning Sickness	Sniff Peppermint. Eat raw ginger or have in a juice. Make massage oil of ginger with olive oil after 1st trimester

More Free Info
www.beautyschoolbooks.com.au

AILMENT REFERENCE CHART

Ailments Reference Chart - Aromatherapy Essential Oil

Methods Are: Massage Blends, Smell Therapy and Vaporizing

Ailments	Essential Oils To Heal	Ailments	Essential Oils to Heal
ABRASIONS & SKIN CUTS	Rose geranium, Frankincense. 1st Bathe in salty water.	GROWING PAINS:	Chamomile, Lemon,
ABSCESS Cold	Chamomile, Lavender, Thyme, Garlic	HAY FEVER,	Hyssop
ABCESS Hot with pus	Chamomile, Juniper, Lavender, Tea Tree but with care	HEADACHE: plus aura headaches	Chamomile, Lavender, Lemon, Peppermint
		HERPES.	Geranium, Lemon
AGEING SKIN	Avocado, Clary Sage Frankincense, Geranium, Rose	HYPOTENSION:	Hyssop, Rosemary, Sage, Thyme
ACHES	Ginger, Frankincense, Peppermint	HYSTERIA:	Cajuput, Chamomile, Lavender, Rosemary
ALLERGIC SKIN RASH	Chamomile, Lavender, Melissa, Rose Geranium,	IMPOTENCE:	Aniseed, Cinnamon, Ginger, Juniper, Onion, Peppermint, Rosemary,
ALOPECIA & BALLDNESS	Lavender, Sage, Onion, Thyme	INDIGESTION,	see DYSPEPSIA
ANTISEPTICS	Boronia, camper, Cinnamon, Eucalyptus, garlic, Juniper, Lavender,	INFECTIONS, VARIOUS:	Eucalyptus, Garlic, Lemon, Onion, Pine... in fact all the essence are
ANXIETY	Basil, Chamomile, Lavender, Marjoram, Thyme	INFLUENZA:	Chamomile, Cinnamon, Cypress,
ARTHRITIS	Black Pepper, Garlic, Ginger, Juniper, Lemon, Marjoram, Thyme	INSECT BITES AND STINGS:	Basil, Cinnamon, Garlic, Lavender, Lemon, Onion, Sage, Savory, Thyme
ASTHMA	Aniseed, Cajuput, Eucalyptus, Garlic, Hyssop, Lavender	INSECTS, TO REPEL:	Lemon (ANTS): Clove, Lavender, Lemon
BED-WETTING,	Lavender- In Diffuser In Bedroom. Sniff Bergamot In The Morning.	ITCHING:	Vinegar,
BITES, ANIMAL:	Eucalyptus, Lavender, Add 1 Dop In 1 Teaspoon Of Olive Oil	LICE:	Cinnamon, Eucalyptus, Clove, Geranium, Lavender, Lemon,
BLOOD PRESSURE High-	Lavender, Neroli, Marjoram, Ylang ylang,	MEASLES:	Eucalyptus (is prophylactic = a preventative of disease)
BLOOD PRESSURE Low	Hyssop, Rosemary, Thyme,	MEMORY, LOSS OF:	Basil, (coriander), rosemary
BRITTLENESS (NAILS):	Lemon, Rose	MENOPAUSE:	Chamomile, Cypress, Sage
		MENSTRUATION, DIFFICULT:	Juniper, Ginger, Peppermint, Lavender
BRUISES,	Ginger, Frankincense, Peppermint	MENTAL FATIGUE, MENTAL STRAIN;	Basil, Clove, Lavender, Onion, Rosemary, Thyme
BURNS:	Chamomile, Eucalyptus, Geranium, Lavender, Niaouli	MIGRAINE:	Aniseed, Basil, Chamomile, Eucalyptus, Lavender, Lemon,
CHAFFED SKIN:	Clary Sage, Geranium, Frankincense, Lavender, Lemon,	MUSCULAR PAINS,	Ginger, Black Pepper, Peppermint
COLDS	Inhalations Of Hot Water And Lemon Oil.	NAPPY RASH,	Use Carrier Oils Do Not Add Any Essential Oils Until Baby Is 1 Year
COLD SORE	Bergamot, Eucalyptus, Lavender, Tea Tree.		
CONJUNCTIVITIS:	Chamomile,	PMT	Learn to meditate. All citrus oils Pls Chamomile. See menstruation.
DIABETES:	Eucalyptus, Geranium, Juniper, Onion		
DIARRHOEA:	Chamomile, Cinnamon, Geranium, Juniper, Sandalwood	SEDATIVES: Sleep Disorders	Chamomile, Clarysage, Lemon, Lavender,, Marjoram, Patchouli
EARACHE: Or Buzzing in Ears.	Cajuput, Garlic, Onion.	STOMACH PAINS, vomiting	Peppermint, Ginger
ECZEMA:	Chamomile, Hyssop, Sage Use Same Method As Dermatitis.	THRUSH (APHTHAE):	Most Oils
EPILEPSY:	Basil, Cajuput, Rosemary, Thyme	TINEA:	Tea Tree
FATIGUE	Rosemary, Juniper, Sniff Bergamot	TONSILLITIS:	
FEVERISH STATES:	Eucalyptus, Lemon, Sage	TOOTHACHE:	Clove
GASTRITIS:	Lemon		

Only add 1 to 2 types of essential oil in Olive oil. Put 100ml of olive oil in 100ml size dark glass narrow neck bottle, add a total of 50 drops of essential oil for body. FOR FACE only add 25 drops . Or in 1 tablespoon of olive oil just add 1 drop of one of the chosen essential oils. Always check the contra-indication of each essential oil. Never ever drink essential oils, add to food and never apply undiluted to you skin.

This information was produced by Clinical Aromatherapist Robyn Ji Smith of Beauty School Books
https://beautyschoolbooks.com.au

Watch Movies That Make You Laugh.

CONTRAINDICATIONS CHART

Essential Oil Contraindications Chart

Contraindications	Avoid-Do Not Use
Alcohol more than 3 drinks	Clary Sage
Antidote To Homeopathy Remedies:	Eucalyptus, Peppermint, White Camphor, Black Pepper
Asthma	Avoid oils high in 1,8 cineole Eucalyptus globulus and radiata (Eucalyptus globulus; Eucalyptus radiata), Helichrysum gymnocephalum, Laurel Berry. Laurel Leaf (Laurus nobilis), Niaouli ct. 1,8 cineole (Melaleuca quinquenervia ct 1,8 cineole), Saro (Cinnamosma fragrans), Ravintsara (Cinnamomum camphora ct), Tea Tree.
Babies under six months	Avoid all essential oil and scented products Unless prescribed by Doctor or certified practitioner.
Bleeding Strong menstrual flow	Basil, Cedarwood, Fennel, Clary Sage, Myrrh, Marjoram, Sage, Peppermint, Thyme.
Blood Pressure (Hypertension per = high)	Eucalyptus, Peppermint, Rosemary, Thyme, Sage, Basil (all varieties)
Blood Pressure (Hypotension po=low)	Lavender, Clary Sage, Melissa, Marjoram, Ylang Ylang, Lemon.
Blood thinners medications Aspirin Warfarin And Barbiturates	1,8 cineole containing oils Ravintsara, all Eucalyptuses, Rosemary camphor/ 1,8 cineole, Cardamom, Helichrysum, Laurel Leaf, Myrtle, Spike Lavender) should not be used with barbiturates. Methyl Salicylate (Birch, Wintergreen), Peppermint and Eugenol (Clove, Basil ct eugenol) Citrus Oils
Cardiac Fibular	Peppermint and Rosemary Thyme essential oil.
Epilepsy	Basil, Eucalyptus (Globulus, Radiata & Polybractea), Fennel, Peppermint, Rosemary, Sage & Thyme.
Estrogen Patch Wearer:	Avoid Geranium, Clary sage, essential oil.
Gastric Problems:	Avoid Cinnamon, Clove and Oregano essential oil.
Inhalations, Douches, Enemas	Cajuput, Cassia, Cinnamon Bark, CO2s, Costus, Clove Bud Elecampane, Fennel, Origanum, Pine, Resins and Savory, Tea tree, Thyme,
Insomnia:	Avoid - Peppermint, Basil, Lemon Verbena essential oil and Rosemary essential oil.
Lactation: - Oils that interfere or dry up milk flow during Lactation	Clary Sage, Peppermint, Sage (blocks the milk duct)
Liver, Kidney & Urinary problems	Avoid Juniper Berry essential oil, Eucalyptus essential oil and Black Pepper essential oil.
Medications - Barbiturates A therapist must prescribe suitable oils to use safely.	When on medications avoid all Citrus essential oils, citrus fruits. & citrus juices for 4 hours after taking medication.
Mucous Membrane Irritants	Thyme, Cajuput
Pregnant.	Basil, Cedarwood, Fennel, Clary Sage, Myrrh, Marjoram, Sage, Peppermint, Thyme.
Puberty In Males- May increase breast size	Lavender, Tea tree all varieties.
Sensitive Skin	Basil, Cedarwood, Cypress, Eucalyptus, Fennel, Lemon, Lemongrass, Lime, Peppermint, Pine, Tea Tree, Thyme, Ylang Ylang
Spa Baths	Avoid Massage & all Essential oils until 30 minutes after spa
Sun and Sun Lamps - Photosensitive to some skin types.	Lemon, Lime, Orange, Verbena, Tangerine, Mandarin, Bergamot, Angelica, Lemongrass, Grapefruit.

Aromatherapist Robyn Ji Smith www.beautyschoolbooks.com.au

It is import that you read these charts before using essential oils. This book copy of the charts may not be as clear to read as you need them to be. These charts are now on my website. https://beautyschoolbooks.com.au/safety-chart

SMELL THERAPY

When inhaled, the scent molecules in essential oils travel from the olfactory nerves directly to the brain and especially impact the amygdala, the emotional center of the brain

Smell Therapy & Happiness Aromas

Purpose – Gain Better Feelings	Oils to Sniff or Add To Your Diffuser
Sad Feelings	All Citrus Oils
Relaxation & Anxiety	Patchouli, Lavender, Frankincense, Clary Sage
Neuralgia & Headaches	Frankincense, Chamomile
Study Fog	Sweet Basil
Memory Loss	Rosemary
Morning Sickness & Energy Loss	Peppermint, Lemon,
Elevate Mood & Increase Vitality	Lavender, Sandalwood, Ylang Ylang, Sweet Orange
Cold, Flue Nasal Congestion	Eucalyptus, Lemon
Revitalize	Lemongrass, & All Citrus Oils - Meditate Then Sniff

As recent as 1980s Doctors have been studying the possible cures for cancer with essential oils. They are powerful healers when administered correctly. Be sure to follow the blending tables and check the contraindications charts above.

- ## Jean-Claude Lapraz, M.D.
  - Consulting physician for Hôpital Boucicaut Surgical and Oncology Clinic, Paris 1989-1996
    - Developed adjunct phyto-aromatherapy treatments for cancer patients to increase the efficacy of their classical treatment while helping to limit side effects
  - Created a curriculum for natural healing taught in numerous countries throughout the world
  - Together with his colleague, Dr. Christian Duraffourd, developed the endocrine theory of terrain which evolved into a new approach to medicine called endobiogeny

CANCER PREVENTION CHART

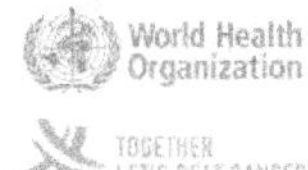

Ways to reduce your cancer risk

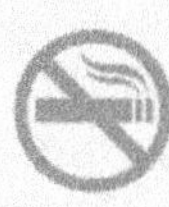
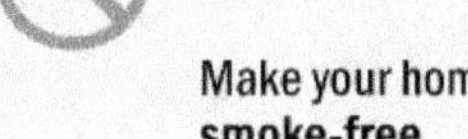

Do not smoke or use any form of tobacco

Make your home **smoke-free**

Enjoy a **healthy diet**

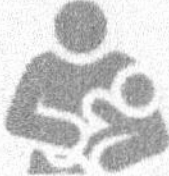

Breastfeeding reduces the mother's cancer risk

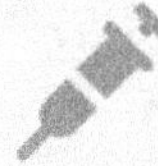

Vaccinate your children against Hepatitis B and HPV

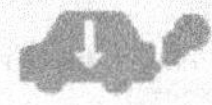

Avoid too much sun, use **sun protection**

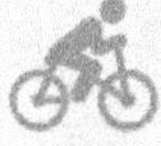

Reduce indoor and outdoor **air pollution**

Be physically active

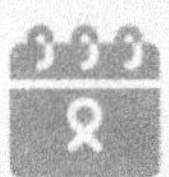

Limit alcohol intake

Take part in organized **cancer screening programmes**

Food For Cancer

PRESERVATIVE FREE SAUCES AND FLAVORS.

This is one of the best dishes you can give someone with Cancer. However, if you have the time learn to make this sauce with raw chilies and raw garlic. They should have a raw beetroot juice with this meal. You can add the beetroot juice to other types of juice to make it more palatable.

HOMEMADE TACO SEASONING MIX

Yield: Enough to season about 15lb. or 7 Kilo of ground meat

Prep Time: 5 minutes

Total Time: 5 minutes

Storage Time; 12 months

Store in an air tight jar in a dark cool cupboard.

INGREDIENTS:

Dried herbs and spices: -

8 tablespoons chili powder

6 tablespoons paprika

6 tablespoons cumin

4 tablespoon turmeric

2 teaspoon garlic powder

Half a teaspoon cayenne pepper

DIRECTIONS:

1. Whisk together all the ingredients in a small bowl.

2. Store remaining seasoning mix in an airtight container at room temperature.

Watch Movies That Make You Laugh.

USE AS TACO MIX

Over medium heat, brown 1 lb. or 500 grams of ground beef and drain. Add 2 tablespoons of seasoning mix and three quarters of a cup water to the ground beef. Simmer, stirring frequently, until the sauce thickens and coats the beef, and there is not much liquid left. To help this food go down more easily add some good quality coconut cream and juice of one lemon. If you want to add a green vegetable add either boiled spinach or peas.

Mum Is Still With Us

As I write this it is September 2009 and we still have mum. She has not had any test done while on the organic healing program, as she wants to leave her life in Gods hands. However, as her Cancer is in the stomach the throat and the bowel but we still have her and look like having her for this Christmas as well. I am very sure the turmeric and beetroot and lavender from Tasmania has done the trick. I do not know if it has actually cured her of Cancer but, it has helped with her energy levels and cleansed her system. It has definitely given her a better quality of life until she meets her maker. She is gardening again and having outings. People are amazed at the colour of her skin and how well she looks and sounds. Mum has not fainted and claims to not be in any pain. Mum is also sleeping all night and is awake and energetic all day long.

Prior to this organic treatment, mum was just sleeping most of the time and vomiting several times an hour. Losing massive amounts of weight, passing out often, and in a lot of pain. Mum had no desire to eat as it hurt and she would vomit.

This turmeric and beetroot diet gave her back her skin tone, energy, stopped the severe pains,, fainting fits and her appetite returned.

Mum and Alisha returned to Woy Woy. Alisha rented out her house and moved in with my mother. Alisha went to the Doctors with my mother and insisted that they do something. Alisha is not the kind of person that you say no to. Because they felt amazed at mums' recovery they operated on my mothers throat so she was able to swallow more easily but explained to Alisha that this was just a band-aid. Mum also had Cancer in the stomach and there was nothing that could be done. They still never gave mum a CT Scan. Mum returned to her Tuesday and Sunday meeting but handed the reins over to someone else.

Naturally the operation on her throat helped. We were told it would not be a permanent fix as she still had the Cancer. They just did something to help keep her throat from closing. That was thanks to my daughter being our family squeaky door. I give you this information with my love and hope it helps someone you love.

Cancer Scans

IMAGING

Do not settle for an X-ray.

Imaging techniques enable doctors to create detailed pictures of what's going on in our bodies without having to open us up. Here are some of the techniques commonly used to diagnose Cancer.

X-rays are a form of electromagnetic radiation that can be used to take photographs of the inside of your body. X-rays are absorbed by dense materials inside the body, such as cartilage and bone, but not by lighter substances like blood.

CT scans (or CAT scans as they are sometimes called) take lots of different x-ray photos of your body from different angles. These are then put back together using a powerful computer to form a 3D image or a series of pictures of 'slices' through your body. This allows doctors to see exactly where a tumor is

MRI scans (Magnetic Resonance Imaging) use magnetism rather than x-rays to build up a picture of the inside of your body. They can be used like a CT scan to view 'slices' through the body, or can make 3D images of your organs. MRI scanning usually produces a more detailed view of the body than x-rays, so doctors often use it to examine the brain.

PET scans (Positron Emission Tomography) are relatively new technology, and is only available in a few hospitals in the UK at the moment. PET scans can be even more sensitive than MRI and x-rays, and they can show how a particular bit of your body is working, not just what it looks like. Cancer Research UK has been leading the way in developing PET scanning in Europe.

Ultrasound scans use sound waves to build up a picture of the inside of your body.

A few years later my niece was told she had cervical cancer. They gave her radiation therapy and it did more harm to her than good. Hayley reported it was extremely painful and she stopped having radiation therapy. My youngest brother and his family live in London.

I am happy to help with any questions you may have. My help is offered for FREE to Cancer Patients, so please make sure I have all the information I need. Height, weight, age, gender and where the Cancer is. What has been tried so far? Please do not write me a short story. Just bullet points, please. I am a witch doctor not a scientist. I have studied the benefits and the chemical components of essential oils (Aromatherapy) at Naturecare College and I have a passion for research. My niece, my cousin and my Aunty went for Chemo and radiation therapy and had a terrible journey and died within a few months of starting treatment.

Because my mother chose the natural way over traditional medications, I only have a small idea about what can work. I am not claiming that this will work for everyone. I would love to hear from people that chose the natural way. You are our future. The Doctors had wiped their hands from my mother all she had was me and my homemade cure.

I pray that this mixture helps you or someone you love the way it helped my mother. You will be able to read the full story when I release the book.

Turmeric And Pepper Tablets

Turmeric cost about $1.50 per pack

The empty capsules cost about $14 for 200 they come in colours or clear.

Wear gloves when filling the capsules with the black pepper and the turmeric.

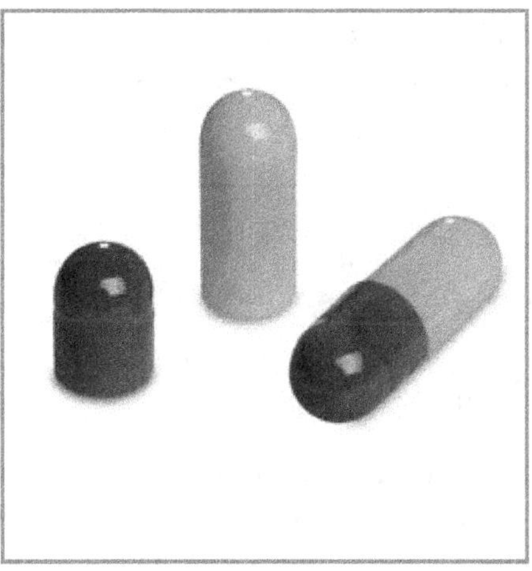

To one50 gram pack of Turmeric add 2 pinches of ground black pepper. This will fill about 50 to 70 capsules.

Put this mix in a small bowl.

Put gloves on.

Watch Movies That Make You Laugh.

Open the capsule and add the Turmeric and pepper mix and reseal the capsule.

Store in a glass jar, in a cool dark cupboard.

You can also add the turmeric and pepper into coconut oil. Put the mixture into piping bag. Allow to cool and set firm. Then pipe into small tablets. These need to be kept in a jar in the refrigerator.

Dose Of Juice And Tablets

Every two days juice three large raw beetroots. Keep in the refrigerator. Add 3 tablespoons of beetroot juice to a glass of other juice. Take 3-4 Turmeric capsules 3 – 4 times a day with the juice.

 Also, the Chinese have some great fixes for Cancer have a look at their information sites. However, you cannot use Chinese cures and have Chemo therapy as they work against each other.

 Do not fear this Witch Doctor cure, it cannot harm you. It restored my mothers quality of life. She went from looking like a dead person walking with no energy to a healthy-looking woman full of energy.

 The other point is Chemo cures some people because it kills off the Cancer cells with poison. It is best **not** to eat herbs and fruits for twenty-one days after your Chemo treatment.

 Email me at beautyschoolbooks@gmail.com

My website https://www.beautyschoolbooks.com.au

Watch Movies That Make You Laugh.

Reiki Meditation And Chakras

When we heard mum had been ill for eight years before we found out, we asked her why she felt she could not confide in us. Mum replied

"Words are very powerful I did not want it to get worse. As you know, I know how to self-heal."

This was true but to carry the load with her would have been the right thing to do. My mum - As a child was taught hands-on-healing and practiced it all her life. This form of healing is now known as reiki.

Mum and her family always meditated daily. To them it was as important as cleaning their teeth. Dad said, on their honeymoon her best friend came to stay the first few nights and when they both started meditating, he found that interesting, but when they started to chant he wondered what kind of girl he had married. Mum was a young virgin and nervous about being in a bedroom with dad. To hear dad, tell that story always made us laugh.

 Reiki is easy to learn and I am happy to teach you if you don't know how. Meditation has amazing benefit. Chakra balancing is mind lifting and a wonderful way to manifest a healing mind body and soul..

I know now, mum was in serious pain for years, but she was dealing with it energetically. Mum said, her morning and afternoon swim also eased the pain. I had noticed when we were travelling she was floating more than swimming. Yet I never thought to question the change.

A Note On Swimming

It is best to do so in ocean water if possible. In the creek or mouth of a river, at the opening to the sea, where the water is clean and calm. If this is not possible for you or the person you love that has cancer swim daily in a pool. Cold water will help with lowering the blood pressure and inflammation, and purifies your skin Warm water soothes the pain.

Keep a check on their or your temperature. When they have a high temperature, a cold-water swim will lower it. A High temperature and indicates a fever which usually means an infection of some kind. Increase their vitamin C and give the person an inhalation.

REDUCE FEVER OIL BLEND

Here is a massage oil to reduce fever. But check the contra indications chart above.

 In a narrow neck glass bottle add

100ml olive oil

20 drops eucalyptus oil

5 drops orange oil

7 drops of clove

1 drop cinnamon oil

Massage into their body twice daily.

Clove oil potent anti-inflammatory properties can help also ease any of the aches and pains associated with a fever. In addition to its antibacterial and anti-fungal properties that kill off all the germs, the antioxidants in clove oil help rid the body of dangerous free radicals so strengthening the immune system.

How to use clove oil for a fever: Make a cold compress by steeping a wash cloth in a bowl of cold water with 30 drops of olive oil 5 drops of clove oil and peppermint oil. Place the cold wash cloth on your forehead, replacing it with a fresh one every half an hour. A cold compress on the back of the neck also helps to reduce overall body temperature.

Never diffuse essential oils while pets and young children are in the house. Be sure that the diffuser is double glazed.

Electric pulse diffusers turn essential oils into toxins so do incandescent lights.   Make sure incandescent lights are off when diffusing essential oils.

Fragrant oils are like poisons to our breath. Always buy pure essential oils from chemists and health food stores. Most are not trained in essential oils and some shop keepers do not understand the difference.

SELF-HEALING REIKI HAND POSITIONS.

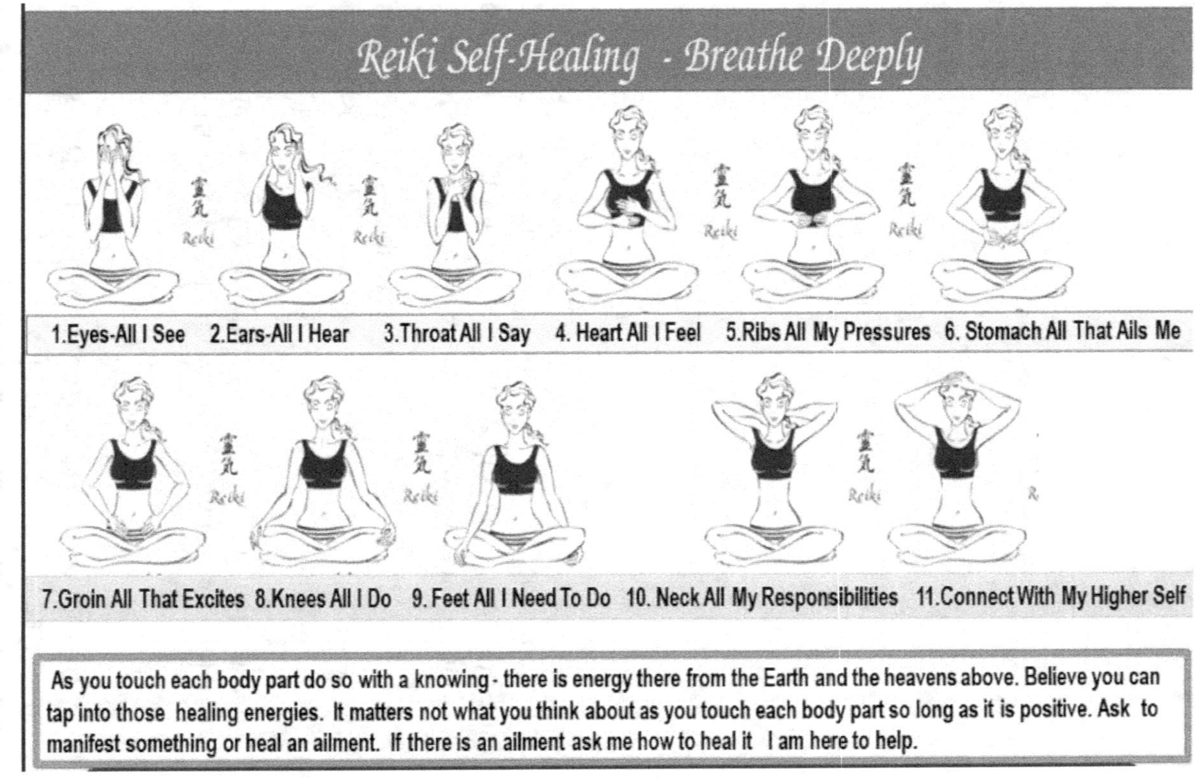

As you touch each body part do so with a knowing - there is energy there from the Earth and the heavens above. Believe you can tap into those healing energies. It matters not what you think about as you touch each body part so long as it is positive. Ask to manifest something or heal an ailment. If there is an ailment ask me how to heal it I am here to help.

Watch Movies That Make You Laugh.

MEDITATION

Meditation works by relaxing the body, increasing awareness, and activating different brain centers. It can help with anxiety, pain, depression, and other negative emotions. It may be more effective with social support or guidance. It affects the nervous system that regulates stress responses. Until you research and learn several forms of meditation.

Start this way.

Take a deep breath in.

As you breathe out sing "OM' ooooommm

Repeat a few times, several time a day.

After The Cure

I am now adding a section here long after mum has gone to heaven. Mum got to the point that she no longer wanted to take the cure prescription. She said, it was her time to go.

As I stated above when mum was told to say her goog byes, I asked her did she really want to go. She said yes I feel it is my time. Mum was eighty-one years of age when she first said that. Then at eighty-four she repeated that statement.

My grandchildren were older and I said to my son, I need you to find someone else to take the children to school. Mum has decided to stop with the organic healings, I need to go and stay with her. Mum wants Alisha to go back to work before she goes.

AFTER MUM STOPPED THE ORGANIC CURE.

Watch Movies That Make You Laugh.

It was January 2011. Mum seemed fine for a few months after she stops using the turmeric and pepper tablets, the juices and essential oil mixtures. Then one night in March I woke to a loud noise. Mum had passed out in the bathroom and hit her face again on the basin. I called an ambulance, while mum was in hospital, they gave her a blood transfusion. When I picked mum up, her doctor set up a morphine drip and showed me how to administer the morphine. He organized a nurse to come daily to help me with mum. Suddenly mum could not cope with us touching her. My brother in London sent over a pair of foam filled lambs wool gloves. They helped us to turn mum over in bed.

Alisha returned to a full-time position, on the same day her dog had puppies. A few weeks later Mum picked up one and said, " this is my favourite". Mum, called her Blossom and we still have blossom. A sweet natured very cute, dog.

Mum was very thirsty and over the last couple of weeks she could not sit up to get her drink. I found myself sleeping in small doses. I would go into mums room often to give her a drink. She no longer could stand hot drinks. I downloaded all the songs her and dad would dance to and played them to her. Over the next few weeks, she became weaker. Alisha went to my sons in Queensland for a few days break before she started her new job. My sister-in-law sent an ambulance and the police to take mum to hospital. I was in shock. Mum had always said she wanted to die at home. As they were putting mum into the ambulance mum called out for me. I rushed to her and she asked why this was happening. I said,

Mum you don't have to go.

My bother stepped in and ordered the ambulance to take mum.

Watch Movies That Make You Laugh.

I asked why he was doing this and he said, Julie (his wife) feels mum would be safer in hospital.

I did not want to argue in front of mum. I comforted her and said, I'll meet you at the hospital mum.

I also did not want to upset my daughter so I told no one what had happened. The next day they put mum into a nursing home.

Two things I noticed.

1. When they were putting food in her mouth mum was spitting it out into a tissue. The nurses aid was chat, chat ,chatting, and not paying any attention to mum. The nurse looked at the bowl and said,

Oh, she has ate it all. That's good. And off she went.

I was flabbergasted. I went to the kitchen to explain what had happened and asked for them to make mum a smoothy. They said, she could not have one she might choke. They came in with a thick substance that mum hatted. I tasted it and it was revolting.

2. Then an hour later they put mum on a shower bed to shower her. I wanted to wash mums' hair. But they insisted they do it.

That was a painful experience for both mum and I. Again, the nurses aid was chatting like she had a motor mouth. She was hosing over mums face and ears in the most uncaring way. I pushed into the small bathroom and put my fingers in mums ears and said

Can you be more careful. You have flooded her ears with water and she cannot breath you are flooding her face nose and mouth. The nurse said

I have been doing this for years she is fine.

So, I turned off the water and told the nurse I would complete mums shower.

A short time later a supervisor came in and started to address me down. I walked out of mum's room and the women followed me. I said,

Please do not address me down in front of my dying mother. Her last few weeks should be all joy and I explained my concerns of the nurse's incompetence.

I asked for her to arrange an ambulance so I could take my mother home. She spoke

I would need to speak with the doctor.

I rang my mothers doctor and he said I would need to speak with the doctor at the nursing home. But, if you do organize for your mother to come home call me and I will come around as soon as possible.

The nursing home doctor refused to allow mum to go home.

The next morning I picked my daughter up from the station and told her how unhappy I was with mums treatment at the nursing home.

When we got to the nursing home Alisha asked mum was she happy to stay there or did she want to come home.

Mum said, No I will stay here I feel safe and do not want to be a burden nor upset Maurice and Julie.

Alisha said, this is your life nan do not worry about how Uncle Moc and Julie will feel. You are no burden we love you.

Watch Movies That Make You Laugh.

Mum said, ok that would be lovely. Can we go now?

I packed my mother belongings while Alisha organized an ambulance and told the head staff what we were doing. They said they would not release mum until her account had been settled. Alisha said

 Maurice has my mums bank cards he will have to pay.

The ambulance came about two hours later. The nursing home made mum sit in a chair in the waiting room. That was another disgrace in our opinion.

Mums doctor came with a nurse to help us settle mum back into her bed in her home and organized nappies and medication. Thy explained to us how to feed mum, bath her and what to expect over the next week or so. What to do when mum passed and so on.

Her nurse and doctor came daily. Spending those two final weeks was not as traumatic as you would think. It was a blessing being able to care for mum. Once you come to terms with the fact that they are going to meet their maker, it is actually, rather blissful. Staying awake is not hard either. Mum was constantly thirsty so I could not have a deep sleep during those final weeks. I certainly felt lethargic. My son and his eldest daughter arrived on the Thursday as did mums older sister and her sons. A friend of my mothers came on Easter Saturday and told Alisha and I to go have a coffee or a swim. When we said to mum we'll be back soon do you need us to bring you back something she said

No. I haven't seen Clare yet. The power of words. When Alisha and I returned Clare was there and an hour later mum passed away.

Clare was a young mother with two daughters. Mum had helped Clare give up alcohol and drugs. My son had gone home on the Saturday morning. He returned the following week with my nieces and their family for the funeral.

Neither of my brothers spoke to me at the funeral, nor did they come to the wake. I was too numb to care.

Family and friends helped me pack mums belonging and give to the St Vincent de Paul's shop.

One other thing you might need to understand is when a person dies at home you need to contact the Paramedics on 000 in Australia. I did not know that, I called mums doctor and he wrote the death certificate.

He told me -who to call to arrange for mum to be picked up. He said

There is no rush. Take your time saying your good bye

So, we spent time washing mum and dressing her beautifully. Close family and friends came to say their good byes. Then a day or so later the doctor returned to ask why we had not organized for mum to be picked up.

I said,

You said there was no rush.

He immediately organized it for me and contacted the funeral service people.

Later that night men arrived in a white van. They tried to put mum in a black bag I became hysterical. As did my daughter. Their van had shelves and other bodies in black bags on the shelves. To think of my mum leaving her home packed in a black bag was horrifying. After they calmed Alisha and I down - they agreed to put her in the bag with the zipper only pulled up half way. Now you know it is a very unpleasant moment in your grieving process. Plus you are not of a sound mind at the time.

After mums funeral service we went on the ferry with all her flowers and the ferry driver stopped east of Lion Island to allow us to float the flowers and say a few words.

Then a month later I went on the Manly ferry to pour mums ashes in Sydney Harbour. Mum did the same with her parents' ashes.

For your reference knowing where to stand is important I had no knowledge of the procedure. Mum said she wanted her ashes to float out to sea. So as we passed the opening (known as Sydney heads) to the sea. I opened the container to pour her ashes over board. Most of the ashes blow back into the ferry and went all over the passengers

After releasing the ashes, I needed to sit down. A man came up to me and said,

Those ashes went all over me and everyone on the deck.

I finished saying my prayer and looked at him and said.

Oh! I am sorry, but you have just be blessed she was a wonderful person and very spiritual. Something amazingly wonderful will happen to you all.

When you are grieving there are many moments of pure joy and you most certainly do some stupid things.

Every wish my mother had for her finale had been done according to her wishes.

May I also say to nurse a loved one at home is life changingly wonderful. Those final weeks mum and I had a very deep connection.

When I was younger and mum said please do not put me in a nursing home I want to die at home She went on to explained some of the horrors she had witnessed during her mum then her dads final days. I said,

Mum, I don't think I can change nappies or wipe your bum when you need me too.

I now know they do not seem to have a bad odour probably because they are not eating solid food. Changing her nappies was easy.

I am grateful that I cared for her at home and will cherish that moment in time forever. The biggest reward from this organic healing will be as it was to me. Seeing them heal and spending perish time with them as they are going through there final days unafraid. I am also blessed to have a daughter like Alisha.

Organic cures do not kill cancer they arrest it. Once you give up so does your body.

I know I have not written this well - because it is a hard topic to write about. But you have the recipe try it.

Love and blessings Robyn.

~~~~.***.~~~~

Other Books At Beauty School Books

Healing and Training Manuals

Foolproof Aromatherapy
~~~~

Watch Movies That Make You Laugh.

Essential oils can heal sooth and energize. Learn how to mix. When not to use and all the benefits for hundreds of ailments listed in alphabetical order. User friendly.

The Antique Healer
This is a much large Aromatherapy book with photos and more healings. Also contains wise old women's remedies.

Positive Spiritual Affirmations
Daily verses to keep you thinking in a wonderfully peaceful positively happy state of mind. Some verses have been composed by the author and other verses are by the great minds of yesteryear.

Dog Care & DIY Organic Medications.
There are many times you will not be able to afford a vet and sometimes when you cannot get to a veterinary clinic. This book will assist you where and when possible to heal your dog in those situation.

<u>**How To Training Manuals.**</u>
Body Piercing Basics
All the main points on body piercing. Correct tray set up and procedures.
Anatomy For Body Piercers
All Body Piercers should understand the body and how it works this is a wonderful tool for any Body Piercer.
Eyelash Grafting Training Manual
Step by step instructions with video tutorials.
Eyebrows Shaping And Tinting To Suit Face Shapes
Step by step instructions with video tutorials on eyebrow shaping, eyelash and brow tinting.
Cosmetic Tattoo Permanent Makeup Micro-Pigmentation Training Manual
A step-by-step training manual. You could actually teach yourself the trade as these books are so well written. The books were tested on students that either live in remote areas and students wanting to learn from home the feedback from them has been very positive.

An Angel For Cosmetic Tattooists
A helping hand for a cosmetic tattooist.
Hair Extensions Training Manual
Learn to create hair wefts, weaves, braids, wax in, and clip in Hair Extensions. There are videos to watch in the eBook.
Supernatural Books:-
Spell Folklore
A great book on how to do some positive affirmations also called spells.
Tarot Scrolls 0-22
Ask a question open a page and an inspiring answer will be there for you to read.
 Numerology Basics
Numerology basics guide you through your birth force vibrations and your seasons of life. It is a short to the point book. Work out who you are and what you should be doing with your career in a heartbeat.
Children's Books: -
Romeo and Juliette Keep Mark Antony
A wonderful story about a puppy born on a boat. His white cute and fluffy. True story with a dash of magic added.
Mark Antony Marries Lizy and Has Puppies
Loaded with photos of all the dogs and the new born puppies. A true story with a dash of fantasy added.

BY ROBYN JI SMITH

Design & Perform Cosmetic Tattooing, Micropigmentation: Follows International Training Standards Sibbsks504a (Beauty School Books)
Alluring Study Of Aromatherapy -For Healers & Perfumers: Follows International Standards For Applying Aromatic Plants SIBBBOS505A (Beauty Pathways Elective Studies 3)
DIY Chakra Balancing: The Art of Connecting To Your Higher Self (New Age by Beauty School Books)Part of: New Age by Beauty School Books Robyn Ji Smith
Chakra Balancing version 2 - Robyn Ji Smith
Learn Perfume Creating - With Natures Gifts: Organic and Alcohol Perfumes Edition 2 (Beauty School Books Training Manuals (For Beauty Pathways Academy) by Robyn ji Smith
Learn Perfume Creating -With Natures Gifts: Organic & Synthetic Edition 4- (Beauty Pathways Academy) by Robyn Ji-Smith

Watch Movies That Make You Laugh.

Learn Reiki Energy Healing version 2 -Robyn Ji Smith
Learn Reiki & Chakra Balancing by Robyn Ji Smith
Got It: Inner Peace (Beauty Pathways Academy) **by Robyn Ji-Smith**
Sustaining A Positively Happy Mind -Loaded with positive verses and affirmations

Diaries & Log Books

Diary -Moon Moods Gratitude & Affirmations

Diaries

Mindfulness and Gratefulness Diary: Edition 3 with Meditation
Diary- Moon Moods -Gratitude & Affirmations
Gratitude and Gratefulness Diary
Blood Pressure Log Book. With charts to keep track of blood pressure, Your pulse & body temperature.

Our YouTube Channel.

https://www.youtube.com/channel/UCbH-MBFfJDSlBqgnRzZ06hQ

Reiki Video 1
https://www.youtube.com/watch?v=m8E5akEl2ho
https://www.youtube.com/watch?v=m8E5akEl2ho
Learn Perfume Creating Video 2
https://www.youtube.com/watch?v=3m_FSsQqWfQ
Learning to create Organic Perfumes Video 1
https://www.youtube.com/watch?v=oKDUNYbuWmg&t=1165s
Blending Essential Oils for lotions Video 2
https://www.youtube.com/watch?v=kVnkQv0kdOI&t=1589s
Learn Body Piercing
https://www.youtube.com/watch?v=Bk3qOFvSa7w&t=10s
Learn Cosmetic Tattooing
https://www.youtube.com/watch?v=2bAuFf6D1OQ&t=14s
https://www.youtube.com/watch?v=iVFutf2sKP4&t=78s

Watch Movies That Make You Laugh.

https://www.youtube.com/channel/UCbH-
MBFfJDSlBqgnRzZ06hQ
https://www.youtube.com/watch?v=O8YqQiwwVHM&t=9s

You may contact the Author

~~~ *** ~~~

JOIN MY FREE REIKI HEALING GROUP
GOLD COAST AUSTRALIA

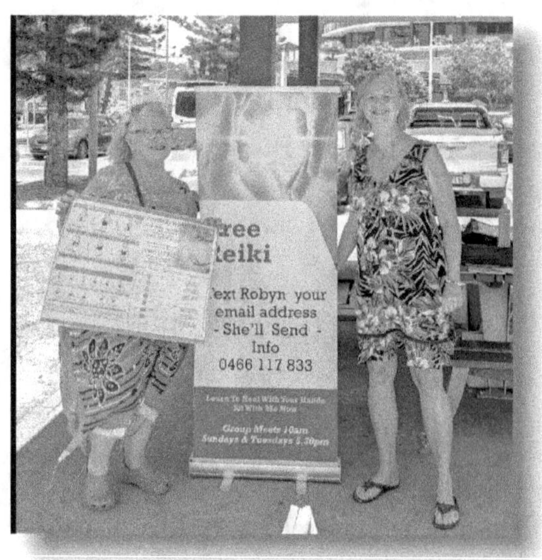

I am on the left and my lovely friend , on the right
Kim helps me help others.

Blessings Robyna

~~~~~.***.~~~~~